THE HARDEST TEST

THE HARDEST TEST

Scott Quinnell

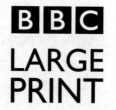

BBC
LARGE
PRINT

First published in 2008 by
Accent Press
This Large Print edition published
2008 by BBC Audiobooks by
arrangement c/o Pollinger Ltd

ISBN 978 1 405 62238 7

Scott Quinnell would like to thank
Karl Morgan for his assistance in
writing this book

British Library Cataloguing in Publication Data available

Printed and bound in Great Britain by
CPI Antony Rowe, Chippenham, Wiltshire

Chapter One

The morning of 21st November 2000 should have been the happiest moment of my rugby career. We were preparing to face South Africa at the Millennium Stadium the following Saturday. As I was eating breakfast, Graham Henry, the Welsh coach, came over to talk to me. An injury had ruled out stand-in captain Mark Taylor and he was offering me the Welsh captaincy for the first time.

I was very honoured and obviously happy. To captain your country is the pinnacle of any player's career. But the more I thought about it and what the responsibility entailed, the more I began to worry.

For the week leading up to the match, I hardly slept. Believe me, it had nothing to do with captaining Wales in front of 72,000 people, nor

1

indeed anything to do with rugby at all. What absolutely petrified me was the prospect of having to speak in front of the players, their families and dignitaries after the game. That was it, nothing more.

My mind would go back to being eighteen again when I was asked to open a fête in my old primary school and the fear that had triggered. Then, too, I hardly slept during the nights leading up to the event. It might seem crazy—I only had to say 'I declare this fête open'. It must seem surprising that something so easy could cause me such anxiety, but my experiences up to that point had left me with little or no confidence when it came to such things.

*   *   *

There's a picture of me when I'm very young at primary school wearing a red rugby jersey. I think it must be one of my dad's, because it's drowning me, but I look very happy. And yet at that time I had no idea what rugby was, let alone how much of a role it would play in the rest of my life. It makes me smile just to look at it.

I started school aged four. Five Roads Junior School was barely 300 yards from where we lived and was very much part of the small village where I grew up.

Learning at that age is all about fun and you soon forget about being left at school every day by your parents. To me, it was just somewhere else to spend time with the friends who were so much a part of my life outside school. That's what made things easier, I guess— we grew up discovering new things together and it was like one big family.

Everywhere there were familiar faces. I recognised the teachers from around the village and even the

3

dinner lady was my best friend Martin's mother—her *cawl* was one reason for *anyone* to want to go to school!

You hear of schools struggling these days with large classes; at Five Roads we benefited from the extra attention that being in small school groups allows.

Thinking back, and with what I know now, I must have shown early signs of learning difficulties. But I don't think there was anything particularly different about me. I was quite a confident kid, eager to have a go at anything.

I remember vividly being given the responsibility of being milk monitor, a job I took to with relish—my proudest moment up 'til then, with the added incentive of being able to have an extra bottle now and again!

Five Roads was and still is very much a close-knit community; everyone knew each other's families and it was safe for us kids to play out until all hours.

Regular events like the carnival brought the community even closer together. I've a vivid memory of one such carnival enjoyed by myself, my friend Martin and my younger brother Craig. We all dressed as rugby players and insisted on walking round all day in those thick, cotton jerseys in the sweltering summer heat, getting up to no good in Mervyn Davies-style headbands. Craig and I had little idea that in the years to come we'd be spending quite a lot of time running around in kit—though I must say I've not been tempted to adopt my godfather Mervyn's 'John McEnroe' look any time since.

*   *   *

The move from primary up to secondary school is enormous for any child. It's gut-wrenching to be separated from the friends you've grown up with and to move away from the security of a school where the teachers know you almost as well as your parents. Leaving Five Roads School was no different—and I really wasn't prepared for the struggle that secondary school would bring.

Chapter Two

My next school was Graig Comprehensive School down in Llanelli itself. I used to catch the bus from the village square just outside The Stag's Head with my friends each morning but, instead of spending all day together, as soon as we got to school we'd all have to go in our different directions.

Arriving at secondary school can be an isolating as well as a daunting experience—for a start it's the first time in your life your academic ability is truly measured, and by being put into streams or sets you get labelled. I found this particularly difficult.

I've always liked the idea of learning and, looking back, I think how great it would have been to be one of those people who could devour all the new information.

Unfortunately, I just couldn't. My poor concentration made this impossible.

I was keen to make an impression, but it wasn't long before I began to fall behind. It was very hard to deal with the fact that while my friends were doing well I was slipping to the bottom of the class. I couldn't understand why, even though I was trying all I could to keep up, I still kept falling further behind.

I tended to keep myself to myself in classes, not wanting to attract attention to the fact that I was struggling. I'd sit at the back waiting for the moment when the bell would ring and I'd be back out in the yard with my mates, where once again I could get involved.

The teachers tried everything to help—looking back I realise how frustrating it must have been for them to work with me, one week, to the point where I seemed to grasp some aspect of a subject, only to see me return the following week with little or no idea of what we'd gone through previously.

I was to learn later that this inability to retain information is one of the key signs of a learning disorder like dyslexia. My short attention span meant that much of the lessons was spent staring out of the window, daydreaming or counting the bricks of the building opposite. Maths was the only subject I grasped to any extent. In others I just kept repeating the same mistakes over and over again.

I'd find things like copying text from a blackboard very difficult. I now know that it was my dyslexia which caused my eyes to jump around the board or the page of a book, meaning I'd miss sentences. This meant having to read things several times, so I was much slower than everyone else at completing the tasks.

One of the major things I

remember is feeling sick at the thought of being asked to read out loud. It terrified me—all the more reason to keep a low profile. Some teachers shouted at me, calling me lazy, and the constant rows upset me very much.

It is important to understand that back then little was known about learning difficulties. I really don't blame the teachers—I guess they had exhausted every method they knew, to little reward. But I couldn't understand why I was being punished. Slowly I began to realise I had problems of some sort. The fact that the other children seemed to move on easily left me feeling very alone. Soon, I was bottom of every class—that's if I was in the class at all!

My wife Nicola remembers finding a box full of my school books from this time when we moved in together, all the pages empty save for the date and the title. That about sums it up, I guess.

* * *

My parents began to realise that things weren't going well. There were the concerns of teachers in the form of reports and letters in the post. I'd often get home from school in tears and lock myself in my bedroom. They found it hard to understand why their eldest son, who had been so full of confidence, was becoming increasingly withdrawn. I used to ask to go to friends' birthday parties, only to quickly change my mind when we arrived, and have to be dragged in by my mother, and then leave soon after. My learning difficulties were now affecting every aspect of my life.

* * *

At fourteen my problems were getting out of control. I'd get increasingly frustrated with myself and got into a fair bit of trouble—if I could get kicked out of a lesson or miss one completely, all the better. I once even punched a friend after a minor argument, breaking his eye-socket in the process. Something had to give.

Despite all this, my parents were brilliant, spending lots time with me while I was doing my homework and trying different tutors to help me along. They looked at every possibility. When they saw that their efforts produced little improvement in school they started questioning themselves, as well as the credibility of the (very many) tutors in the Llanelli area who were assigned the huge challenge of improving my grades!

As my father has since said, 'We knew he wasn't *twp* or dull, but it was frustrating.'

I was pretty sharp when it came to things like sport but a complete failure academically.

*   *   *

Eventually my parents came to what I suppose, looking back, was a natural conclusion—that it was the sport, particularly the rugby (which I had by that time begun to get heavily involved in) which was to blame.

They imposed the ultimate penalty on me, stopping me playing rugby at Under 15 level—it turned out to be the only level I didn't play at.

I was devastated. By this time, rugby was all I really wanted to do and although I saw the importance of education I found it impossible. Everything seemed to be against me.

Thank goodness the ban didn't last for long!

Chapter Three

What's in a name? I was born Leon Scott Quinnell on August 20th 1972 in Morriston Hospital, Swansea— the wrong side of Loughor bridge as far as my family and future was concerned (though I'm told I was quickly rushed over to the Llanelli side in order to take my first breath!).

My father Derek had been a three-times British Lion as well as a Welsh international, and he had the honour of being the only player in the Lions squad not to have already been capped by his country when he went on the tour to New Zealand in 1971. My uncle is Wales and Lions legend Barry John and my godfather Mervyn Davies also pulled on both the Wales and Lions jerseys. (No pressure on me then, whilst growing up, to pick up the oval ball!)

Rugby did seem to be everywhere, even with my mother—she'd become a massive fan of the game after years of following her brother, Barry, and of course my father. My two youngest brothers, Craig and Gavin, followed us into the game as well, becoming professionals in their own right. So it's not hard to imagine what the topic of conversation was around the dinner table when we were growing up!

At the age of eight, I began showing an interest in the game which would eventually become my life. I asked my father to take me down to Stradey Park, Llanelli, to play for the U11s.

It might sound surprising, but up to then I hadn't really sat down to watch a game of rugby, not even to watch my father. I know now that my learning difficulties meant I didn't have the attention span to watch a whole match. In honesty I'm still not one for watching the game, though watching the game is now what pays the bills!

*   *   *

I recall my father being away a lot playing rugby when we were young. In 1977 he was on tour in New Zealand for three and a half months and again in South Africa for the same amount of time in 1980.

As well as our good friends in Five Roads, we were lucky to have Nan and Granddad next door to us, which must have really been a help for my mother when Dad was away. It was great to have an extended family right there. My grandfather Stan would spend hours with us as kids. I loved it when he helped me make bows and arrows and, later, encouraged me to drive diggers and tractors. What more could a boy want?

While on tour, my father was only

allowed one phone call home a week and whenever I got to speak to him I spent the whole time in tears. In the end my mother decided that she would relay messages between us—a lot less trauma all round!

*   *   *

It had been Mr Rees, a lovely teacher at Five Roads School (who went on to teach both my daughters, Samantha and Lucy), who initially planted the rugby seed. He was the first guy to actually encourage me to pick up a rugby ball, taking us all training.

Although Dad must have been quite pleased when I showed an interest in the game, it's important to say that he never pressured me to follow in his footsteps. He was more than happy for me to make my own way in the world.

People often ask me about my hopes for my son Steele. I think they expect me to say that I'm longing for him to follow in my footsteps. That couldn't be further from the truth. I may be proved wrong but I think Steele is more likely to paint a game of rugby or write about it than play in it, and so be it! As I've learnt from my father, all you can do is let children follow their own paths in life.

*   *   *

Being on the rugby field brought on an instant change in me. Failure to deal with school had made me more and more withdrawn, but having the ball in my hands, caked in mud, seemed to bring out the real Scott. I felt in control for once and at last began to feel the rewards of effort and practice which had yielded so little at school.

At other times I could be found on my bike on the hills around Five Roads or playing cricket or football with friends: anything as long as it was sport, exercise and fun. The more involved I was in sporting activities, the more my confidence grew.

Later the family moved down to Pen-y-fai Lane, and the new house had the advantage of being near to town, and overlooking Stradey Park. I began to take a real interest in watching Llanelli play, and I was also now nearer to the weights gym and the squash courts. It was in these places I began to spend much of my time.

I've learnt that people with learning difficulties develop what they call 'coping strategies' to deal with their condition. It usually means involving yourself in things that you are good at and not exposing yourself to unfamiliar situations, I guess it's because of fear of failure.

As books and writing and general academic work became more

difficult for me, I began to spend more and more time on the rugby field or watching the game and, later, working out in the gym. It was where I felt comfortable, where I felt a real sense of belonging.

I still see that sense of camaraderie as rugby's ultimate appeal. Wherever I've been in the world through rugby I've always felt a part of a family. This was no different in the early days.

*   *   *

As I made progress in the game, I started to feel sure that it was what I wanted to do for the rest of my life. After a few games representing the school, I was made captain, which was a massive honour for me. I also began playing for Llanelli schoolboys and went on to captain the Under 16s on tour to St Helens—my first ever trip away from my parents and a truly memorable occasion.

Whilst there I got to meet former Llanelli great Roy Mathias and also Stuart Evans (whom my dad had coached for a time with Wales). At sixteen I was 6' 1' and a bit of a lump but Stuart literally had to come through the door sideways to meet us! It was incredible—he's one of the biggest men I've ever come across in the game!

On the Sunday we got to see St Helens play at Knowsley Road and I was able to witness for the first time the wonderful sense of occasion that is part and parcel of the 13-man game.

After the match I was taken to meet the Saints' board, who out of the blue offered me a place in their academy set-up. I found it hard to believe what I was hearing. It was an incredible compliment and of course a real boost to my still fragile confidence.

But I felt very much that I wanted

to make my mark in rugby union, and at that time my only wish was to play for the Llanelli first team. Everything else could wait.

*   *   *

Back at home, things were much the same. I began to miss school regularly, Wednesday afternoons in particular, which I would spend training. I recall one teacher cornering me one day and saying, 'Quinnell, you'll never come to anything playing rugby, boy!'

His advice had come far too late for me!

I began to show even more dedication to the game. I'd recently had a major eye-opener and a narrow escape, just missing out after a Welsh Under 15 trial, where I played at prop! I'd put on weight and was never so glad to have a hammering in my life! I realised if I was to get away from the dreaded front row and have a future in the game, I really had to focus.

Thinking about it, my negative experiences in school may have made me even more determined to prove myself. I wouldn't say I was a natural, but I was fortunate to have inherited a physique which, with work, helped me ply my trade in the No. 8 position.

Playing for Llanelli youth at sixteen, week in week out, against older boys of eighteen and nineteen really served to toughen me up and get me into shape. Believe me, you take some big knocks, but if you want it badly enough, you're always there the next week, ready for the next bout!

My career was moving at quite a pace and I had little time to stop and think about education and the problems of the past. Besides, I had found something rewarding. I felt useful at last.

I wonder sometimes whether or

not that teacher has followed my career—I haven't bumped into him since!

Chapter Four

By the time I was seventeen I had more or less given up going to school. My time now was split between rugby and working for my dad as a representative in the family company. But somehow my father managed to persuade Graig headmaster Dennis Jones to allow me to stay enrolled in school. I had to re-sit maths in order to remain eligible to compete for a Wales Under 18 cap as well as work part-time for Dad. The re-sit was a minor diversion, keeping me in school longer than I'd anticipated—but I was prepared to do anything to pull on that Welsh jersey! I'd turn up at Graig in my Escort 1.4 company car (yes, I was a boy racer too!) wearing my school tie and leave later having changed into my work clothes and tie.

That Welsh U18 trial soon came around. It was held at Aberavon's Talbot Athletic Ground and was a huge moment in my life. I began the match in the 'possibles' team, the mission being to play my way into 'probables' for the second half. I was really determined to take this opportunity to show what I could offer. And sure enough, at half time, I was told to change sides for the rest of the game and to carry on where I'd left off, this time in the colours of the 'probables'.

Next it was back into the clubhouse for sausage and chips and the longest two-hour wait of my life. When the announcement finally came and my name was read out, it was like all my Christmases and birthdays had come at once. I was to pull on the cherished Welsh jersey against the Scots.

*   *   *

Memorably, I played for the Welsh Under 18s team against the Welsh Youth at Stradey Park. It was not memorable because we beat our senior opponents, but because the Youth team that day contained a certain Neil Jenkins and Scott Gibbs. That result would supply valuable ammunition for the future!

Then I was off to New Zealand with the school team, where we became one of the only sides (junior or senior) ever to win all six tour matches. This was no mean feat in the land where they live and breathe rugby almost as much as we Welsh!

The fact that I went on to miss my final maths exam, because I was conducting a different kind of maths involving my father's company and a business deal in Swansea, shows where my priorities now lay. I was chasing a different dream entirely! I didn't have time to feel that bad.

Not that my father had gained a top class employee. Working for him showed how my learning difficulties affected my life in the real world, as it had done at school. All employees were required to fill out call sheets and time sheets. When it was time for mine to be given in, I usually made some excuse, like I'd left them in the back of the car. My father's secretary Sue was probably the only reason I managed to keep on top of things. She would help me fill out the order forms at the end of each day and make sure everything was in order.

*   *   *

The highlight of my time with the Welsh Youth came in a match against England in Blackpool, where I somehow managed to score four tries in a big win. On the opposite side that day was one Lawrence Dallaglio. Thinking back, I wish I'd made a bit more of that victory. Managing to get one over on 'Lol' in a Welsh jersey only happened on one other occasion, on a famous sunny day in 1999—but more of that later. I guess I peaked too early!

1990 was a very busy year for me. I represented Wales in Canada at Under 19 level and played for Wales at Youth level.

Then came my big chance. Llanelli were looking for youth players to join members of the first and second teams to play away at Penygroes in their centenary match.

I was given the nod. I cannot describe how great it felt to pull on the jersey for Llanelli for the first time. Remember, I had turned down an invitation to play league at St Helens just for this moment. I was following in my father's footsteps and representing the place that I loved. I really don't remember who won that day, but it didn't matter. I had worn that famous scarlet jersey. I prayed that this was to be the first of many occasions that I'd have that honour.

Chapter Five

The following season, 1991/92, brought with it another big opportunity. Llanelli's success domestically meant a number of our big name players, such as Lawrence Delaney, Phil May, Phil Davies, Emyr Lewis, Rupert Moon and Tony Copsey, would be away serving Wales in the World Cup. I was invited up to the first team. This was it. It was the massive opportunity that I'd been waiting for.

As well as myself, players such as Paul Jones, Huw Harries and Mathew Wintle, who had toured Canada with me at Wales Youth level, were also called up. On top of that, Allan Lewis, who was now coaching at Llanelli as Gareth Jenkins's no. 2, had been our coach at Wales Under 19s level. This all meant that even though I was moving on to a new, massive challenge, I had people around me I was familiar with. This helped a lot.

In the October of 1991 I met my future wife Nicola in a Llanelli pub one evening. I knew instantly she was the one. I recall very early in the relationship being on Llanelli beach together when Nicola began showing me over and over the correct way to pass a rugby ball (her dad Bryn coached Bynea Rugby at the time). I was bemused but said nothing.

A few days later she rang me after seeing my picture in the local paper. In one of the most surreal conversations I've ever had, she told me, 'You play rugby for Llanelli!' To which I replied, 'I know. Where do you think I go every Monday, Wednesday, Thursday and Saturday?' She said, 'Oh well, I thought you just worked out in the gym like my brothers!' That's what I love about Nicola—she's never really been a rugby fan. She used to watch me play firstly for the social life and secondly to see that I didn't get hurt. It was a good thing I always drove home!

We soon moved in together and it was not long before we had our first child, Samantha. It was a wonderful time, like a whirlwind: I didn't want it to stop. I was still working for my father, which helped make ends meet in those pre-professional days but between that and training and playing at the weekend, I found I had little time left to spend with my new family.

*　　*　　*

I'll always remember seeing my first live Cup Final. It was 1985 and Gary Pearce converted a late drop goal to beat Cardiff and win the Cup for Llanelli. It sent real shivers down my spine. The whole of Llanelli seemed to be in Cardiff that day and being there was superb.

And to think that by the end of that busy 91/92 season, I myself was lining up in a Cup Final singing the National Anthem along with players such as Phil May, Ieuan Evans, Rupert Moon, Mark Perigo and Ricky Evans!

What a moment it was, knowing my friends and family were there in that massive crowd. We went on to defeat deadly rivals Swansea 16-7 that day, which topped things off nicely!

* * *

You often hear of sports men and women having superstitions when preparing for a game. For instance, they may put their kit on in a certain order or listen to a certain song to get 'psyched-up'. It was around the time of that Cup Final that my lucky underpants entered my life.

I had worn these pants when playing all season. I'd developed a close bond with them, so much so that the thought of appearing in a match without them was unbearable.

On the day of the final my wife Nicola, mother, father and brother Craig had gone down to Stradey to catch the bus to Cardiff, as is the tradition for our supporters.

I was left at home to finalise my preparation and pack ready for the big match. I loaded my kit-bag as usual, but to my horror my lucky pants were nowhere to be seen! I decided quickly that either my father or Craig must have put them on. I rushed down to Stradey with a spare pair to catch the bus before it left. Luckily it was still there, so I boarded and demanded to see what pants they were wearing. It turned out to be Craig who was the villain of the piece. I quickly made him change into the spare pair and headed off to the final safe in the knowledge my lucky charm was in my bag. I'm certain we would have lost that day otherwise!

* * *

Playing rugby regularly for my beloved Llanelli in the shadows of the same saucepans on top of the posts that had beckoned my father was a great feeling. Even if the journey distance was much the same to Stradey Park as it had been to Graig (they are barely a mile apart), emotionally and psychologically I had come a long way.

Dad was always around, ready to give me advice on the game and I was never short of role models to look up to in the shape of his former colleagues and team mates who'd become close family friends over the years.

Being born into what's been called a 'rugby dynasty' (a term that makes me cringe) didn't automatically mean my transition into the game was easy. As rugby became increasingly part of my life I quickly learnt that having a name like Quinnell had its negative aspects as well as positive ones.

Some people liked to assume I was only in the Llanelli side because of my name. I sometimes got into scrapes of an evening in town after a match and a couple of pints. After all, I was still a teenager at this time. And I'd be the first to admit I wasn't always in the right. But you're always going to have that in a small town, I guess. I was a big boy, too, and there are always people who want to have a pop to prove a point. But I learnt to avoid certain situations and environments. I began to realise that I needed to sacrifice some things in my life to get on in the game. Fortunately Nicola proved to be a calming influence on me too. We met at the right time.

*　　　*　　　*

It was a similar story on the field. I recall one cup match, when we were due to play Furnace United. Sometime the day before one of the boys had heard that the Furnace players had each put £10 in a pot to be taken by the first man who could get me off the field (presumably on a stretcher) in the game. I was used to the fact that I was becoming something of a scalp, but found this particularly underhanded and decided that even though I was tired (I'd played the night before for Wales Schools against France) I would now definitely play a full game. There was no way on earth I'd leave the field and give anyone the satisfaction (and the £150 quid!). Needless to say, the match was a bloody affair and when the ref blew up I was exhausted, black and blue but more than happy to have lasted the eighty minutes.

The Furnace boys were understandably a bit miffed and not

entirely pleased when on our way back through the tunnel I suggested that, having lasted out, the money in the pot was rightfully mine! Of course, I didn't see any of it.

Chapter Six

If the 91/92 season had been a dream start for me, getting first team rugby with Llanelli and picking up a cup-winner's medal, the season which followed could not have been more of a contrast.

In the October of '92 I picked up a knee injury early on in a match against Pontypool. Unfortunately, through total inexperience, I chose to play on. I came off after the game in great pain, struggling with an extremely swollen knee. Little did I know that this was the start of a long-term knee problem which would ultimately bring about the end of my career.

I struggled on for a few weeks until eventually I was advised to take a little break to rest the knee. This gave Nicola the ideal chance to make an honest man of me.

In September, we ran away to Scotland to get married (with the permission of both families!). It was a very basic ceremony and a quiet affair all round. Nic still reminds me to this day that our wedding lunch consisted of a pasty and a can of Diet Coke each!

I arrived back home happily married, but my bitter-sweet year was far from over. My knee was worse than ever. I don't think I realised at the time the seriousness of the knock. My career could have ended right there. I had badly damaged a posterior cruciate ligament, no minor bump! I was told I needed to fully rest it for two to three months.

What I *did* realise all too well was that it would be an uphill struggle to get my first team place back. Llanelli had players such as Lyn Jones, Mark Perigo and Emyr Lewis, all seasoned internationals, in the back row. It was going to be tough.

November 14th, 1992, saw one of those great moments in Llanelli Rugby's history. The mighty Wallabies, reigning World Cup Champions, arrived at Stradey Park on tour.

In a legendary encounter, Ieuan Evans scored under the posts and Llanelli went on to win the match 13-9. I was in the crowd that day, still nursing that knee. I watched as the pitch was invaded at the final whistle and Rupert Moon was carried aloft by the fans as Delme Thomas had been twenty years before. As a supporter I was delighted but I was also gutted. The realisation that I could have been there on the field that day took the shine off it for me. Nevertheless I was immensely proud of the boys. Little Llanelli had taken on world-beaters again and won. It was a result in the same mould as Llanelli's legendary 9-3 win over New Zealand in 1972. As in '72, the pubs once again ran dry and it was a chance for another generation to say 'I was there', even if they weren't!

To cap a frustrating year for me (though not for the club), I also sat out the Cup Final against Neath. I had played a little, to test the knee, but I was nowhere near fully fit. I was on the bench to watch an improbable drop goal from Emyr Lewis in the dying moments win us another trophy. It was great to be part of a successful squad but, as I've said, I'm not really one for *watching* the game. I really felt I was missing out big time.

*   *   *

I spent that summer working hard with Peter Herbert, Llanelli's fitness advisor. As well as getting the knee back in shape, I also had to work on my weight. It was like my Welsh youth trial days all over again. I didn't want to miss my opportunity to get back into playing for Llanelli when it came around.

That summer I also got a surprise visit from Mike Ruddock, then coach of Swansea. I was flattered when he asked me if I'd consider signing for them for the following season. I explained to Mike that my only aim at that moment was to break back into the Llanelli starting fifteen. After all, I was a Llanelli boy—I'd supported them all my life. I thanked him all the same and he respected my decision. It was a compliment, much like that from St Helens earlier in my career, which made me even more determined to push on and prove myself. Thankfully, the following season would prove to be the best of my career.

After returning to full fitness, the following term saw me regain my place in the Llanelli side. Coach Gareth Jenkins favoured a rotational system during early season, which allowed me, along with the rest of the back row, to get our fair share of game time.

Fortunately I seemed to show enough ability to be selected to play two matches for Wales A that autumn, one against the North (Wales) and one against Japan. Stuart Davies picked up a knock around this time, which was to rule him out for the first team's next game against Canada. I really felt for Stu—he's a great guy—but his injury left a big opening for me; one which I had to take.

I was called up to Sophia Gardens in Cardiff the weekend before the Canada game to train with the first team. I'd played a bit at No. 6 with Llanelli, rotating with Emyr Lewis between that and the No. 8 position. It was there, at blind side, where I was selected to make my full Welsh debut against Canada the following week. The only time I've played in that position for Wales. Heck, I didn't care what position I was picked at. I'd even have played at prop!

When the team was made public I was overwhelmed by all the cards and telegrams from well-wishers, family and friends. Today I guess it would be all e-mails and text messages. It was incredible, a humbling experience. Thinking back, this was the culmination of a lot of things in my life. I'd practically dropped out of school with only my rugby to keep me afloat. Of course I had also been fortunate. I had a young family to support and that knee injury could easily have ended my career before it even got started. But reaching this point was proof for me that I had made something of myself. I'd trained hard and worked at my game, particularly in coming back from injury. In the words of

Thomas Jefferson, 'I'm a great believer in luck, and I find the harder I work, the more I have of it.' (You've even got me quoting US presidents!)

This was it; I was being rewarded for my efforts in something at last. It was a wonderful experience to run out at Cardiff Arms Park in the Welsh jersey that day, even if it was green—it was the three feathers on my chest which mattered. I'd been brought up alongside my father's proud collection of Wales jerseys. Now I had one of my own.

Unfortunately it wasn't one of Wales's better days at the office. We lost 26-24. To add insult to injury, it was Canada's outside half, Gareth Rees, of Welsh heritage, kicking the winning points. But, for obvious reasons, despite the result, that game will always have a special place in my heart.

Chapter Seven

A week later, I had the massive honour of being selected by the Barbarians, the famous invite-only team with a tradition for all-out flowing rugby. It was the custom for the Baa-Baas to select some uncapped players, and it was as one of those that I'd originally been chosen. The only snag was that after the Canada appearance I was no longer an uncapped player. I remember resigning myself to the fact that at least I'd earned that Welsh cap—the Baa-Baas could wait for another day. However, I was surprised to receive a call from Baa-Baas' President Micky Steele-Bodger to congratulate me, telling me I'd been selected anyway, as a capped player. It was Neil Back who would be the uncapped representative. Things were just getting better!

The Barbarians were to face New Zealand in Cardiff. All I can say is that when the match kicked off, I kept wanting to pinch myself. It's not every day in rugby you run out against players you really look up to. I was lining up against people like Ian Jones, Va'aiga Tuigamala, Zinzan Brooke! To have the chance at the age of twenty-one to play against these boys was a dream come true.

New Zealand ended up victors 25-12.

*   *   *

Next it was big-time rugby, as I waited for my call-up to play for Wales in the 1994 Five Nations, that most famous of rugby competitions. When you are growing up in the game, this is *the* competition—any player will tell you that. The Tri Nations may have that southern hemisphere glamour, but the Five (later Six) Nations is the real deal. It was magnificent to be a part of it at last.

We played Scotland first and I'll never forget the driving rain that day. Mike Rayer scored two tries as we trounced the Scots 29-6. Then came Ireland, and another win in a game which was soured by my Llanelli team mate badly breaking his jaw.

When France came to Cardiff, next up, we knew we were in for a difficult ride if we were to maintain our winning run. They were bringing with them a wonderful side packed full of class players such as Benazzi, Sella, Benetton and Saint-Andre. They were possibly one of the best sides in the world at the time.

In the first half I managed to steal the ball at the back of the line-out. We were about 40 yards out (though as the years go by and I tell this tale, it's up to about 80!). I barrelled through a few French defenders and before I knew it I was over in the corner for my first try for my country.

I watched it recently on TV and hardly recognised myself as that young lad. What I do recall, and what's clear on watching it again, is the delay before the realisation hits home that I've scored, and my face lights up. I remember Rupert Moon jumping on my back and Phil Davies around me too, all Scarlets together. It was magnificent. I knew where Nicola and my parents were in the crowd and I made eye contact with them. It was the stuff dreams are made of. We went on to win 24-15. We now had to go to Twickenham to take on England for the chance of the Grand Slam.

*　　　*　　　*

If the French challenge had been tough, we would now be head to head with the biggest pack in world rugby. Our preparation wasn't ideal. We were late arriving at the Old Stand in Twickers because of traffic congestion. It meant we had less time to prepare and get out there on the field. Then I soon realised what being star-struck really was when faced with players such as Ben Clarke, Dean Richards, Dewi Morris, Will Carling and Jeremy Guscott who I'd watched playing for many years for England and the Lions on TV. It was awe-inspiring stuff.

Unfortunately we went on to lose that day 15-8, but still won the Five Nations Championship on points. Memorably, Ieuan Evans went up to collect Wales's first trophy for many a year.

*   *   *

That summer I was away on a tour of Canada, Western Samoa, Fuji and

Tonga with Wales. It was a massive honour to represent my country around the world, but I was also finding it difficult being away from my young family for so long. I came to fully realise what my father must have gone through, leaving Craig and me with my mother to go on tour all those years ago. A day didn't go by when my thoughts weren't with Nicola and Samantha back home in Wales.

On returning home my life was about to take a new twist. The try I'd scored against France was big news. I suppose you could say it put me on the map. That summer the phone didn't stop ringing. Most of the interest seemed to come from up north, from the rugby league clubs.

I was in a bit of a spin. I'd just had the greatest of seasons in rugby union. Perhaps it would be a good time to end on a high. The very thought of changing codes made my heart skip a beat. It would be a massive move not just for me in terms of my career but also for my young family.

Mike Burton, the former England and Lions prop, who would become my future agent and a close family friend, really opened the doors for us in rugby league, advising my father to talk us into going up to speak to Wigan.

Chapter Eight

One Sunday in September my father drove Nicola and myself up to Lancashire. Jack Robinson, the Wigan Chairman, had asked us to wait in the hotel opposite their Central Park ground before the game against Sheffield. He had arranged for one of his directors, Tom Rathbone, to meet us. The idea was that we'd watch Wigan's match that day and have a chat.

*   *   *

We were sitting in the bar on one of the sunniest September days I can recall, surrounded by hundreds of Wigan and Sheffield fans, when in walked a man in a long raincoat, black hat and sunglasses. Nic and I looked at each other; we thought the KGB had just walked in!

As the man approached us, all around Wigan fans were calling him and saying, 'Alright Tom?'

He leant in close to me and enquired, 'Scott?' To which I nodded. In an instant he removed the hat, glasses as well as the coat to reveal a blazer with the biggest Wigan badge on it you'll ever see.

'Ah, I'm Tom Rathbone. I've been sent to get you,' he said and shook my hand.

We had a few drinks and made our way over to the stadium.

As we walked across the road I was greeted by people saying, 'Hi Scott!' and, 'How are you, Scott?' It was all pretty comical. In those days, remember, you could be banned from rugby union if you were seen anywhere near a league match. But Wigan's interest in me, it seemed, was hardly a state secret. It made Tom's disguise all the more hilarious. Thank goodness there were no such things as forums and internet chat rooms back then. I wouldn't have been allowed back over the Severn Bridge, let alone home to Llanelli that night!

Jack Robinson met us and showed us round the stadium which has all that wonderful history attached to it. Wigan had just won the world club championship in Brisbane and had a side full of stars. They beat Sheffield that day.

* * *

My decision to move north to play rugby league for Wigan was not taken lightly. I had been enjoying my time at Llanelli and had of course developed strong friendships both on and off the field. I'd also reached a pinnacle by pulling on the prized Wales shirt, and it was difficult to contemplate never experiencing that sensation again. I had to come to terms with the realisation that I would be saying goodbye to the game of rugby union forever, because in those days the rules dictated there was no going back once the codes had been crossed. I knew as well I'd have to deal with those who I'll politely call the 'traditionalists' who would perceive me as a traitor for moving up north.

But at the end of the day I had to think about Nicola and Samantha who had seen their time with me shrink as my career grew. The move to Wigan meant that instead of spending most of my time outside of rugby working to support my family I was at last able to split my life between rugby and family.

I went up to Wigan alone initially, basing myself in a hotel, though Nicola made frequent visits and we house-hunted together.

I soon began training with the lads at Central Park. It was quite tough being alone, but the training programme took so much out of me,

I don't think I'd have been much company anyway. It was a major step up from what I was used to at Llanelli. As well as having to learn the ropes in a different game, my new employers required me to increase my seventeen-stone frame by another two stone. My first few weeks were spent performing five sessions on the weights (whereas I'd been used to two), eating to refuel, and soaking the aches and pains away in the bath.

Learning to run at speed backwards for the first time in my career was a bit of a challenge, too. It's not as easy as it sounds!

*   *   *

When Nicola and Sam moved up, the first few months in Wigan were pretty strange for us as a family. Just being away from Llanelli was difficult. We were used to having our parents nearby to help out with things like babysitting and there had always been friends around. However Joe Lydon, a league legend, was just coming to the end of his career with Wigan, and he and his wife Nicola took it upon themselves to help us settle in. For this we'll be eternally grateful.

The people of Wigan really live and breathe their rugby, so in this sense it was very similar to Llanelli. If we lost a match at the weekend it would be the topic of conversation and debate in the town for the rest of the week. Their passion for sport helped me feel very much at home, I guess.

I became friendly with two more of Wigan's recent signings, Barry McDermott and Terry O'Connor. Even though we were all competing for similar positions, we supported each other, training hard and generally enjoying each other's company.

Wigan's success meant it was

difficult to break into the first team, but it was very much a squad environment. It didn't matter if you played in the first thirteen or for the reserves—everyone seemed to get along.

*   *   *

I'll never forget my first game against Salford. I was picked for the seconds after being at Wigan for what seemed a very short six weeks.

The plan was to give me a run-out in the last ten minutes to acclimatise to the game and the rules. But our second row tore a hamstring after fifteen minutes and my gentle introduction to league went completely out of the window.

I recall taking the ball up for the first time, after being on for about a minute, and being hit by what must have been about ten to fifteen big forearms. Looking up from the ground, with blood gushing from my nose, I was confronted with the grinning face of Richard Webster, the former Swansea player and another to have crossed codes, who said simply, 'Welcome to rugby league.'

Call me mad, but I actually enjoyed the experience. I think it put me in good stead for my time up north.

Chapter Nine

It was a midweek fixture away at Doncaster which brought about my full first team debut.

It was hard to believe I was lining up at second row in the same side as Andy Farrell, Dennis Betts, Martin Offiah and Jason Robinson—true legends of the game!

I lasted about five minutes. Perhaps the occasion was all too much for me, or I clumsily ran into the elbow of an opposition player! Either way, I soon found myself dazed on the ground after being hit once, getting up and playing the ball the wrong way, and collapsing again. The next thing I knew I was at the side of the pitch in the arms of the physio who was busily attending to my broken nose.

At half time Wigan coach Graham West came to see how I was doing, which I thought was very kind of him. Groggily I told him I was feeling a little better and that at least my nose had stopped bleeding. 'Great,' he said. 'Get back on for the second half.'

That's the difference in the two games: in rugby union the bang on the head would have sidelined me for three weeks by law. Here, I found myself back on the field before I knew it, even though I felt like I'd been run over by a bus. It was certainly a test of character.

I don't know if the Doncaster boys had a pot on me that day, but, like the Furnace boys before them, they too would have walked away frustrated and out of pocket. Even though playing on wasn't my choice this time!

*   *   *

Later that season I was asked by Wales rugby league boss, Clive

Griffiths, to attend a training session and later to watch the forthcoming international against Australia. The Welsh team that day featured the likes of Allan Bateman, Dai Young, Rowland Phillips and Paul Moriarty —players I was already familiar with. If I had any doubts about the physicality of league, this game was to well and truly get rid of them.

You could almost feel the big hits from where you sat. As a measure of the sheer brutality of the match, John Devereaux got taken off with a broken jaw. But if any one thing stood out for me that day it was the performance of the colossal Mal Meninga. What a player—he had the sublime skills to match his sheer force. If he represented rugby league at its best, I knew I had my work cut out!

*   *   *

I have lots of great memories of my

time at Wigan. I got the call to represent Wales rugby league at the 1995 World Cup. We had one particularly brutal encounter against Samoa at the Vetch, Swansea. The game had to be delayed because of the massive crowds—many people had to be locked out. As you can imagine, the atmosphere was electric. Samoa were so physical that if you gave less than 100% commitment, you could be sure not to last the eighty minutes in one piece. I'll never forget Allan Bateman desperately looking through the grass for his tooth after one big hit. We won that day but unfortunately lost to England in the semi-final. I scored four tries against arch rivals St Helens on Boxing Day 1995.

*　　　*　　　*

Leaving Wigan was tough. We'd been made to feel at home there as a family and I'd developed a great affection for its passionate and knowledgeable rugby fans. But the word had come from Mike Burton (who was now my agent) that Richmond were interested. The rules on players crossing codes had been relaxed, allowing me to move back to union. Jack Robinson, the Wigan chairman, said he'd be sad to see me go, but honestly admitted Richmond's offer was a good one for Wigan as well as for me.

To make my decision even more difficult, I'd just been selected for the preliminary Great Britain rugby league squad to tour Australia—a massive opportunity. The ultimate for any British league player. A lot to give up.

But on the plus side, the British Lions Union Team were due to tour South Africa in 1996. Making the move back to union now would give me a good opportunity to work towards that goal. If I wanted to follow in my father's footsteps and become a Lion, it was now or never.

Saying goodbye to Wigan we found ourselves once again leaving friends and a real support network behind. Wigan and its people had been good to us.

Finding ourselves in Richmond, in the 'big city', had an instant negative effect on both Nic and me. It was a difficult place to live. We were small-town people at heart. We found London very cold and impersonal.

The move down to Richmond coincided with the birth of our second child, Lucy. For Nicola it was a difficult pregnancy. A caesarean was required. I'll never forget the doctor offering to bring the birth forward to allow me valuable time to be with them before I had to travel to Scotland for a match. He later asked for free tickets and I duly obliged. A small price to pay for what he'd done.

Richmond were a second division side, but were desperate to succeed in the premiership, and had made a number of big signings in the process.

Whilst there, I was soon joined by many familiar faces—Allan Bateman, Barry Williams, John Davies and my brother Craig all signed up. It became a bit of a joke that we were turning into Richmond Welsh!

It should have been a great time. I always thrived on having familiar faces around me. But in reality I spent the first few months wishing I'd never made the move.

One of the key factors was playing in the second division. Yes, it was a new challenge for me but I was used to big crowds at Llanelli, Wigan and for Wales, and missed this at Richmond. Also, the club's big spending meant that our star-studded team was expected to win comfortably each week. I had always thrived on the buzz of a good battle. Sadly, these were few and far between and it was difficult to remain motivated. I'd worked hard to get where I was in the game. This ethos had helped me through the tough times. Now at Richmond I felt like I was going through the motions. It left me increasingly disillusioned, depressed and unhappy.

Richmond were eventually promoted to the Premiership, which was great, but the magic of the game was no longer there for me.

I'm eternally grateful that Richmond came calling for me when they did. They allowed me the opportunity to get back into rugby union. But by this time I'd had enough. I would soon be getting a call of a different kind, back home.

Chapter Ten

The 1997 British and Irish Lions tour was the major reason I left rugby league.

I was still at Richmond when I got my chance to go on the South Africa tour. Allan Bateman and myself both got called up to the squad. I'll never forget the day we received the letters. It was April 2nd, my daughter Samantha's birthday. The kiddies party we'd arranged turned into a massive celebration. I remember the bouncy castle we'd hired being taken over by the adults after the kids gone to bed. A great time was had by all.

It's difficult to express what a Lions call-up means to a player. Growing up, I had my goals, to play for Llanelli and to play for Wales. I didn't really look beyond that. But the Lions is something else. As an international, you get used to playing against the other home nations but to come together as British Lions is magnificent. I'd left rugby league for this opportunity, and when it came it exceeded all my dreams.

We had a week's preparation in London under the management team of Ian McGeechan and Jim Telfer. The camaraderie was instant. Despite our wide range of personalities, we knew we were all in it for the same thing and it was bigger than all of us. Though it was odd at first to be playing alongside people you'd usually be in violent opposition to on the field!

There was one anxiety. I'd been suffering with a double hernia in the build-up to the tour. But I received two cortisone injections and it was decided that these, coupled with a dose of strong painkillers, would see me through.

My tour started very well, with me scoring two tries in the first game against an Eastern Province Invitational side.

But four weeks in, with the tour going from strength to strength, I began to struggle. I knew my hernias weren't going to last out.

I recall one key moment. We had a rest day and Allan Bateman, Barry Williams and I decided to go to the cinema to catch a film. As we crossed a busy road, a car sped around the corner and forced us into an easy jog to the other pavement. The pain in my groin was intense. I knew there and then my tour was over.

It was the hardest decision I've ever had to make. But there I was facing McGeechan and the tour party, knowing I was only running on about 70%. I'd left a promising league career for this, only to see my

Lions dream fall short two weeks before the first test. But I knew I couldn't give my all and I've never been one to sell myself or others short. I had to tell them I couldn't continue.

I found myself back home for the remainder of the tour. It was heartbreaking, being once again a spectator, a role I'm useless at. I locked myself in the front room with the TV to cheer the boys on between shouting the plays and set pieces at the screen; the things we'd gone over and over together in training.

Ask any sportsperson—watching your colleagues out there on the field is the hardest thing ever. It was like being back at Llanelli again and watching my pals beat Australia. I felt the elation when the series was won, but the personal disappointment of falling just short of a test cap was intense.

I vowed then that my sole aim

for the next four years was to get that Lions cap in 2001.

Chapter Eleven

New Zealander Graham Henry, 'The Great Redeemer', had taken over as Welsh national coach and I was more than happy to feature in his plans for the upcoming internationals against South Africa and Argentina.

Once again there was a slight problem. I had brought home with me an unwanted souvenir from Richmond. In one of my last appearances against Wasps I'd been sent off for a late tackle on Lawrence Dallaglio. (I'd told the ref that I'd got there as soon as I could but he didn't see the funny side.) In my defence, Richmond went on to claim the tackle was barely a third of a second late. I'll call a 'no comment' on that one!

But the RFU imposed a 14-day ban, sufficient to see me have to sit out the clash with South Africa.

I did what any law-abiding player would do in the circumstance—I lodged an appeal.

The hearing was due on the Thursday before the South Africa match on the Saturday.

The thing is, we'd brought home another souvenir from London, one which was far more welcome. Nicola was expecting our third child.

The birth was due to be another caesarean. Fate determined that Steele was set to be born on the very same Thursday as the appeal hearing was due. I was duly granted compassionate leave, which postponed the hearing a week. This meant I could now play against South Africa!

In a press conference earlier that week, Graham Henry had been asked about my inclusion in the team. To the journalists it didn't make sense to have me down, as they were sure the ban would be upheld. A wily Henry (who had already been prepped about Steele's forthcoming arrival) told the press that it would all be fine, that he'd had a chat with 'the man upstairs'.

So Steele, bless him, like Lucy before him, was involved in the politics of his father's rugby career before he'd even had a chance to open his eyes!

*   *   *

The South Africa match was to be another at our new adopted home, Wembley. Cardiff Arms Park was in the process of being transformed into the Millennium Stadium. It was a wonderful feeling to run out on the pitch that I'd seen my beloved Liverpool F.C. victorious on in so many finals on TV. We went on to lose the game 28-20 on the unfamiliar Wembley turf, but our heroics that day were a sure sign of things to come under

Graham Henry.

His era as Wales coach saw the dragon develop a new lease of life. His appointment had meant a clean slate for Wales and had been an opportunity for different faces to play their way into the squad. He had arrived with few preconceptions about players and knowing little about the club game in Wales.

Although he had experienced pressure, pride and no little success as coach of Auckland, he was yet to understand the Welsh psyche. But by the end of his first Five Nations match up at Murrayfield, where he witnessed 15,000 Welsh fans travel up, I think he was beginning to get an idea of what he'd taken on!

*   *   *

By October 1998 we were back home in Llanelli. I took a big pay cut to return to Wales but, after the misery of London, being home was more than worth it. I guess you have to go away to really appreciate what you have. When we left, four years previously, I never expected to be playing in that Scarlet jersey ever again.

Ironically, my first game back at Stradey Park was not in the scarlet of Llanelli, but in the red of Wales as we ran out 43-30 winners. It was the first of a series of hard-nosed battles against the ever-emerging Pumas that would be played over the next year or so.

Being back in Llanelli was wonderful for the family as a whole. We had left as three and returned as five. Our old friends were still around and we settled back in instantly. What I love about the town is the fact that it really doesn't change. We set up our new home back in Five Roads. We'd come full circle but it also felt like we'd never left.

Returning to Stradey Park was

such an emotional experience. After the lows of Richmond it was great to be back. I felt at home though also strangely restless. I felt deep down that I owed this club. They hadn't had the best of me.

Few clubs inspire the pride and passion of the Llanelli Scarlets. They are up there with Munster, Leicester and Toulouse. When you pull on the scarlet jersey it's a feeling you carry with you forever. The late Ray Gravell, a former president and player at the club, was one figure who embodied that spirit. If you can get close to emulating him, you are getting nearer to the magic. His sudden death has been a sad loss.

I was keen to get cracking with my new career back at Llanelli. I knew there was some way to go if I was to achieve that goal of making the Lions again.

I was quickly back into the swing of things, as were the club. That first season we made the cup final against Swansea at the Vetch. 1998/99 had been Swansea and Cardiff's rebel season. They'd fallen out with the Welsh Rugby Union and opted out of the Welsh league to play friendly matches instead against English Premiership sides.

Being a Llanelli boy through and through, you rarely need motivation to take on the Jacks, especially in their own back yard. But expectations were high for that final. We had the pride of the remaining Welsh clubs to fight for against a Swansea side who had (temporarily) turned their backs on Wales.

It turned out to be the worst final I ever played in. Colin Charvis, carrying a broken cheekbone, scored two tries in a 37-10 demolition.

I'll never forget Scott Gibbs's comment after the match that the game had been 'men against boys'. His superior tone really hurt. It's something which stayed with me. I

would never allow myself to be
outclassed that way again.

Chapter Twelve

The highlight of the 1999 Five Nations was the match against England on that sunny day at Wembley.

I don't think I've ever had as many phone calls from well-wishers before a match as I did that morning, and I remember the ground being packed and joking that Wales must have been deserted that day.

I recall we just about kept ourselves in the game and were awarded a penalty near the end of the match. We kicked for the corner and hoped for a successful line-out. The move from the throw-in was definitely one we hadn't tried before as it involved me passing the ball. I didn't do that often! I remember almost knocking on before shuffling the ball on to Scott Gibbs. He broke away and only had Matt Perry to beat. I shouted, 'Run over him, Gibbsy!' But he did something I'd not seen him do often. In inspired fashion he skipped off his left on to his right, and with one arm in the air, was over the try line.

The Welsh contingent at Wembley went crazy but Neil Jenkins still had to convert the try to win us the match.

I've played on the same side as some of the best kickers in the game: Frano Botica, Jonny Wilkinson and Stephen Jones. But when it comes to the crunch Neil Jenkins would be my choice every time. Jinx, The Ginger Monster—what a magnificent servant to Welsh rugby he has been. That said, I still turned my back on the kick and hoped for the best. The roar of the crowd told me he had done it.

*   *   *

More joy was to follow. We went

over to Argentina and won a series which was certainly not one for the faint-hearted, and came home to famously beat South Africa in the first match in a not yet completed Millennium Stadium.

So, going into the 1999 World Cup, we were on an eight-match winning run. It was a matter of great pride for the Welsh nation to host the World Cup. And as always in Wales, expectations were high.

The opening game at the Millennium Stadium was us against Argentina. I don't think I was the only one who was getting pretty sick of seeing them! It proved to be yet another physical encounter but we managed to come out of it with a win.

We then went on to overcome Japan in the second game.

Third up were Western Samoa. This match will go down as one of the worst games I've played in a red jersey. Trevor Leota seemed to follow me around the pitch all game. When I got the ball there was no way round him and certainly no way over him!

I gifted them a first-half try with an intercepted pass. It eventually went on to help them to a 38-31 victory. But believe me, it was more than our egos which were left bruised and battered after that result.

Despite that shocker, we'd done enough to progress to the quarter finals to face the 1991 champions and eventual winners, Australia. This was a highly emotional and passionate encounter. Looking back, we played so well we really could have won. I think referee Colin Hawke awarded some dubious decisions Australia's way, including their first try which was clearly a knock-on. They went on to win 24-9.

I remember sitting at the dinner that night, pondering over an opportunity lost. The result was disappointing, even if the performance was one we could be proud of.

It was the only World Cup I got to play in, and on home soil too. It goes down as my biggest disappointment in rugby.

*   *   *

Llanelli is renowned for its reputation as a cup side. Their record in the Welsh Cup is second to none. But it was the Heineken Cup which we coveted most of all. It's a competition which to this day brings out the best in us.

I was fortunate on my return to Llanelli to be a part of what became quite an adventure in that competition over the next few years. Two matches stand out for me, one for all the right reasons and one for all the wrong ones.

London Wasps were the visitors to Stradey Park in January 2000. To book ourselves a vital home draw in the semi-finals we had to beat Wasps and win by 10 points.

It was one of those massive cup occasions at totally full Stradey Park. We started at a blistering pace, forcing the Londoners to play to our strengths. We went in 10-0 ahead at half time.

Ian Boobyer was superb that day. The guy was everywhere, really in the faces of the opposition. Even Lawrence Dallaglio, renowned for his chat during matches, began pleading to the ref to shut Boobs up. During one team huddle I was talking to the players and looked around only to find Boobyer missing. I turned to find him on the edge of the Wasps huddle, cheekily advising them what he thought they should be doing! I'd love to repeat his words of advice here, but they are totally unprintable!

We eventually went on to win the match 25-15, with Craig Gillies running thirty yards up the right to touch down to secure the 10-point margin. It was one of our greatest ever Heineken Cup wins.

No prizes for guessing my Heineken Cup low point, though I guess it's the worst of three I could have chosen.

It was at Nottingham's City Ground, which hosted a nail-biter of a semi-final between ourselves and Leicester. In the run-up, Leicester captain Martin Johnson had labelled the fixture 'The Battle of Britain'. Although it never lived up to its billing, it's a game no Llanelli player or fan will ever forget, however hard they try.

In front of a capacity 29,500 crowd we entered the last quarter 12-10 up. As time ticked by I think even Leicester began to think that their reign as kings of Europe was coming to an end.

After what seemed like an eternity of stubborn defensive play from us,

Leicester were awarded a penalty 25 metres out. Their kicker Tim Stimpson was pretty reliable but I recall feeling that with the angle, this was just about on his limit. I noticed he pinched a few more yards when placing the ball and I went up to the ref David McHugh and insisted he take the kick from the right spot. McHugh just waved me away. Stimpson gave the ball a mighty whack and, just as it looked as if it was falling short, it hit the bar, hit the post, hit the bar and heartbreakingly popped over. The ref turned and ran. It was an indication to me that he knew he'd made a mistake. The final whistle went, and Leicester were victorious 13-12.

The manner of defeat really killed me. To play so well and to lose in that way was criminal. I felt so sorry for the huge number of Llanelli fans who'd travelled all that way. I'm told someone had put a sign on the entrance to the M4 at Hendy: 'Would the last person to leave Llanelli please put out the light.' That sums up the humour and commitment of the Llanelli faithful.

Chapter Thirteen

2001 brought a second chance for me as far as the British Lions were concerned. I'm immensely proud of the fact that I stuck to the vow I made in 1999. I'd set myself that goal and overcome some pretty huge obstacles to get there and be selected.

Not long into my second spell at Llanelli I had found out that rheumatoid arthritis had set into my left knee. This made training and playing extremely difficult. I was pretty much told my days were numbered. Of course I was in no way ready to accept this. I had some unfinished business to attend to.

I was fortunate to have coaches such as Gareth Jenkins and Graham Henry in place at the time. They understood my problem and were prepared to look at different training regimes and programmes to keep me going in the game.

I also can't thank David Jenkins, Hywel Griffiths, and later Wayne Proctor at Llanelli and Mark Davies the Wales physio, enough. They knew what it took to keep my fitness up to standard whilst rehabilitating the knee.

I spent a good deal of time in the pool, working with Peter Herbert who'd looked after my knee before. There was also good advice from Wales colleague Rob Howley, who recommended silicon injections which allowed me to run and train harder. The skill and care shown by these people extended my club and international career.

I have no doubt that without them there was no way I would have become a Lion again.

*   *   *

Before I knew it I was in Brisbane

with the Lions and 35,000 British fans. Graham Henry was in charge and I was more than glad that he'd brought Wales fitness coach Steve Black with him. Blackie too was sympathetic when it came to training and he knew exactly how to get the best out of me while taking the pressure off the knees.

I remember being at the team hotel before the first test. My father rang to say he was on his way over to collect some tickets I had for him. After we met, I decided to walk back to his hotel with him, just to get away from the rugby environment for a while.

Little did I know what would face me as we walked into the lobby of the hotel where he was staying! The first person I saw was ex-Wales fly-half Jonathan Davies signing in at reception. Then there was Llanelli legend Phil Bennett sitting chatting to a group of fans from Felinfoel. Next I was called over by a gang from the snooker club back home where I'd regularly call in for a couple of pints after a game. It was hard to believe. Even my Dad's old mate Dai Twin, who I hadn't seen for years, was there; he'd flown over from Hong Kong to follow the tour. It was like walking into a hotel in Llanelli. Wonderful and surreal at the same time.

I'd been trapped in a bubble for weeks. Seeing all the familiar faces brought me down to earth. It relaxed me and I managed a good night's sleep before that first test.

*   *   *

Graham Henry had asked Willie John McBride to hand out the jerseys to the team the next day. McBride had toured with the Lions an incredible five times. He holds the record of seventeen test caps. He also captained the most successful Lions side ever which toured South

Africa in 1974 and won the Test series 4 -0.

His speech was so rousing it sends shivers down my spine just thinking about it now. He told us about the passion of the Lions and what the jersey meant to him. Then he started handing the jerseys out. It was a magical feeling to hear your name called. He seemed almost reluctant to give each jersey away and I'm sure he'd have played in that first test himself if he'd been given the chance. To shake his hand and look him in the eye was almost like seeing a transfer of power from him to you. When the presentation ended I think we'd have killed for him and that jersey.

*　　　*　　　*

The Gabba in Brisbane is a strange old venue for rugby. It normally hosts cricket, so it was odd to see the rugby pitch plonked in the centre of this giant oval.

We warmed up inside, nerves jangling. Captain Martin Johnson said a last few words, but I don't think any of us needed any more motivation. It was wild running out on to the field in front of so many British and Irish fans. They apparently outnumbered the Aussies three to one.

The game kicked off at a ferocious pace with Jason Robinson going over in the corner. Howley was immense throughout the game at scrum half and Brian O'Driscoll showed the Aussies just what all the fuss was about. I even managed to get over from the base of a ruck to score myself. By that time we were up 29-3!

Lots of people still ask me about that try. Well, not so much the try itself, but the nod I did after touching down. They say it's one of their enduring memories of that tour. All I can say is that it was a bit of a personal sign. There, with the ball under my chest on the Gabba turf I'd finally achieved my goal. Everything had come together for me. More than that, it had taken over two hundred and fifty people to achieve that goal. That nod was for all the medical staff, coaches, fellow players, friends and family who'd been there for me when I was down. Without them none of it would have been possible. It was no longer just a personal goal.

We went on to win the game 29-13 but were to lose the series 2-1. All the same, Australia 2001 will always be the stuff of dreams to me.

Chapter Fourteen

It was 2005 and the Llanelli Scarlets were due to face Cardiff Blues in the Arms Park. My knee had been troubling me quite a bit in the run-up to the match. By now it was so problematic that it would just lock completely. Things weren't looking good, but we had some of our internationals away in camp and it was a game we needed to win. I decided at least to give it a go and see how long I could last out. It was to be my last ever competitive game.

At the final whistle I came off the field with my wrist in a lot of pain. It turned out I'd fractured my scaphoid, an injury requiring six to eight weeks out of the game. Between that and my knee it was clear the gods were trying to tell me something. Perhaps if I'd pulled out before the match I might have lasted the rest of the season, maybe even another.

But I was never to pull the scarlet shirt on again.

*　　　*　　　*

After I retired, the WRU. were kind enough to offer me the use of the Millennium Stadium for a testimonial match. I would share the event with Rob Howley, who had also been forced out of the game because of a wrist injury.

The plan was that Rob would put together a World XV, to play a British and Irish XV selected by me. The response from the players was magnificent. Big names like Bobby Skinstad, Mick Gallway, Jason Leonard, Joost van der Westhuizen and even footballer Ally McCoist all volunteered their services.

A few days before the match Stadium Manager Paul Sergeant called Rob and me in. He said he'd had a great idea for our entrance into the stadium. I imagined being driven in on golf buggies or on horseback. Then Paul hit us with his big idea. He suggested we absail from the roof. Rob and I looked at each other in disbelief, but before we had the chance to say anything Paul said, 'Good, that's sorted then.'

*   *   *

Before kick-off, both sides lined up on the halfway line and waited for our entrance. Fireworks went off and we began our descent. It's the first time ever I've been quicker than Rob at anything. Before I knew it, I hit the turf of the Millennium Stadium. I don't think that patch of ground has been right since!

The match itself was an absolute joy. It was great because I got to play on the same side as both my brothers, Craig and Gavin—the only ever time all three of us have been on the same side.

We'd arranged something even better for the last two minutes. My father, who had been team manager, and my son Steele, who was six at the time, came on to the field. It was an extra-special moment. There we were, five Quinnells, all on the same side, all wearing number eight.

We packed down for a scrum on the 22-metre line for the last move of the game. Kieran Bracken fed the ball, my father picked up and passed to Alex King. Steele, who up 'til now had shown little interest in rugby, had positioned himself correctly and took a pass from King. He ran toward the try line, only to be faced by the mighty frame of Salesi Finau.

The Tongan, 5' 10' tall and 5' 10' wide, tried to get out of the way but couldn't. If I'd done what Steele did next, I'd probably be still be playing now. He looked up and passed straight to Finau, who, panicking, threw it straight back. My father and I together picked Steele up and carried him over to touch down and score.

I think after the match Steele signed more autographs than any of us. It was to be the last time I'd ever put my boots on for a match. It was so good to be able to share that moment with my family.

Chapter Fifteen

At school, rugby had been my salvation. It was something I could do which wasn't hindered by my learning difficulties.

It's interesting when I look back now, because I can see the ways in which I consciously and unconsciously dealt with my problems through rugby.

Of course, it helps if you're doing something that you are interested in. Since leaving the game, I've met so many people with learning difficulties who are immensely talented in different fields, whether it be music, art or sport. Like me, they all found an interest and pursued their goal. Many were diagnosed early and coped with their problems whilst focusing on their interests.

But so many have similar stories

to mine. Their schooling was a time when they felt completely isolated. Like me, they found solace in the things that interested them while their education suffered.

*   *   *

In rugby I quickly learnt that any lapse in concentration could result in me getting my head knocked off. That's something that has helped me focus a fair bit! On the park I found it helped to break the game up into small sections to allow me to concentrate on one phase of play at a time. Sometimes it would help to play from whistle to whistle, although this very much depended on who was refereeing the game that day. An open, flowing game might be great to watch, but played havoc with my concentration levels!

As soon as one phase was over I wouldn't dwell on it. Once finished I knew I couldn't affect what had happened, so I cleared it from my mind. Then I would be fresh for the next phase.

As I moved on and the game became more professional, I found myself in team meetings and the like. Unlike at school, I made sure that for these I was right in front. Maintaining eye contact with the coach whilst he spoke helped me to avoid drifting off.

In the latter years at Llanelli I was required to keep a diary, recording my diet, exercise and general thoughts on the game. This was left to Nicola. In rugby as well as outside of it I had support. At Llanelli, if, after a group discussion between the forwards, things had to be written up on the board, Robin McBryde was magnificent. He understood, and would do it for me.

When I had a go at coaching Llanelli after retirement, I was sure never to put myself in a position where I had to write on a blackboard during team talks and training sessions. I was fortunate that the other members of the coaching team, Sean Gale, Kevin Williams and Neil Boobyer, were aware of my problems and stepped in for me.

But as amazing as they were, I guess they were also helping me to hide from my problems.

Rugby had been my ultimate coping strategy, helping me hide from the reality of my learning difficulties. I'd had the humiliation of fans throwing autographs back in my face when I'd spelt names wrongly. But on the whole, I'd coped pretty well. I'd forged a career for myself despite my problem.

Now, out of the game, the reality of my learning disabilities came to the fore. I'd relied so much on others, especially Nicola, to deal with the everyday bits and pieces— paper work, filling out forms etc. Right from week one of our relationship I was asking her to do things like write cheques for me.

I was now pretty much a full-time family man, with all the responsibilities that brings. I was faced with the prospect of making a life for myself and my children outside of rugby. This would involve being invited to make speeches at dinners and presentations, working as a rugby pundit—how many sleepless nights would they bring!? The business world ran on the internet and email—I couldn't even write notes for school for the kids. Nicola deserved a break, too.

Worst of all, we both had to face up to the reality that the kids had begun to show signs of learning difficulties.

*   *   *

The idea that I might be dyslexic had first come about completely by luck. It was back when I was about twenty-one and Nicola, who was an excellent typist, had offered to copy up a hand-written thesis on learning difficulties which her friend had written.

I remember her calling me into the room as she worked. She began to reel off a list of dyslexia symptoms and, to our amazement, I ticked every box. It was all there. The answer (if not the cure) to what had caused me years suffering at school was contained on this one sheet of A4 paper.

Had we acted on it then, who knows how my life would have turned out? But I was so focused on my rugby career at the time I didn't give it much thought. I think deep down, too, there was that fear of being labelled. All the clues were there, but I never allowed myself to be tested for dyslexia officially.

*   *   *

I had now begun working regularly for Sky television as a rugby pundit. In the TV studio before a match I got talking to fellow pundit and ex-Scotland international Kenny Logan. Someone had brought in a piece of paper and Kenny asked me if I'd read it. 'You're kidding,' I said, 'I'm dyslexic.'

Kenny couldn't believe it, and began telling me about the problems he'd had with learning difficulties. We realised we had quite a lot in common. He told me of this treatment he'd just gone through called the Dore Programme. His wife Gabby Logan had seen a programme about it on TV and they'd signed up. It sounded bizarre. It involved beanbags and wobble boards, pretty unorthodox stuff. But Kenny sang its praises. I decided there and then to pursue it. Perhaps it was too late for me, but hopefully the kids would benefit. I didn't want them to go through what

I'd gone through at school. I wanted them to have the opportunities to learn and enjoy that I never had. Kenny passed the number of Wynford Dore, the programme's founder, on to me and I rang him the first chance I got.

I explained to him that I wanted to put the kids through the programme and I told him about my experience of dyslexia. Wynford suggested that it made sense for me to go through the programme, too. I agreed. If I wanted the kids to progress, the least I could do was show willing and go through it with them. It was time I faced my demons.

*　　*　　*

In January 2006, we all went to the Dore Centre in Cardiff to be tested to see if the programme was suitable for us. I was diagnosed as severely dyslexic. My problems were a lot worse than Lucy and Steele's.

One of the key tests was for balance. I learnt that with learning difficulties like dyslexia and dyspraxia, things like co-ordination and eye tracking as well as balance are affected.

'Learning difficulties' suggests problems with reading and writing. It's difficult to make a connection between those and physical activities. But the exercises would work on the cerebellum, the part of the brain which processes information and makes things automatic.

This began to make sense. I had always become easily tired when reading and writing. When I thought about it, I could see how my dyslexia left me having to concentrate much harder just to do simple tasks because nothing was automatic. These were skills that most people take for granted. Obviously my poor eye tracking had been responsible for the way in which my eyes would skip around over a page.

I stepped onto the machine which tests your balance and fell off instantly. I'd been playing rugby since the age of eight—I would never have thought balance would have been a problem.

When we got home and started the exercise regime, Nicola was as sceptical as I had been. I guess it's hard to take sitting on Swiss balls and throwing beanbags in the air seriously as a treatment at first. But when you get into it, you realise how tricky the exercises are.

As I had done with my rugby I began to really apply myself to the routines. I was away a lot with work and had to be sure to take the equipment with me. To get the best out of it takes real dedication. I had to be strict with myself as well as with the kids.

A BBC film crew asked if they could record my progress throughout the year, and I was more than happy if it served to raise awareness of learning difficulties and help people to recognise what people with such problems go through.

After about six weeks Steele was keen to try riding his bike again. It had been heart-breaking to see him fail on his previous attempts, when all the other kids his age were cycling around. I tried to dissuade him, telling him to wait a little while longer, but he was adamant.

I held the seat as he rode. I let go after about ten yards. In disbelief I watched Steele continue, thirty, forty, fifty yards. 'Dad, don't let go,' he eventually shouted. 'What do you mean?' I said. 'I'm back here.' He had no idea he was on his own.

I've played fifty-two times for my country but never been as proud as I was that moment. That day proved to me that the programme was working and it gave us all the belief to push on.

That summer we were on holiday in Lanzarote. At the airport on the way out I bought a couple of books. I started reading the first on the plane and to my amazement I finished it after three days. By the time the week was over I'd read both. I can't begin to express how this made me feel. It's something that most people take for granted. I'd never before managed to get through a book. My eyes would start to hurt, or I'd give up because the words would jump all over the page.

Over the next few months I read more and more and even began going on the internet and writing e-mails myself for the first time. It was an emotional time as I began to realise all the things I'd missed out on over the years. But at least I knew that my children wouldn't be missing out.

They too were progressing all the time. They brought their school reports home and sat with me as I read them. Just to think—when I was at school I'd do all I could to hide my reports from my parents! I couldn't believe the change. They had both improved in all subjects and the teachers were amazed with their progress.

I could see them coming out of themselves, too. They had always been happy, but they were really starting to grow in self-esteem. It was a great feeling for the family as a whole.

When I returned to Cardiff in the December for my last test I wasn't prepared for the results. I'd begun the year in the lowest 5% for reading and writing. I was now being told I was above normal in those areas. I broke down. I had excelled at rugby. I was used to being patted on the back and congratulated for things I'd done on the field. But this was something new. I'd gone through school being called a failure, so much so that I'd begun to believe it.

Now I was being told I had succeeded. I had overcome dyslexia. I never thought it would feel so good to be normal.

Today I'm asked to do as many talks on my experiences with learning difficulties as on my rugby career. For the first time ever I actually enjoy going to school, where I speak to the children. It's been a remarkable couple of years. I now represent the Welsh Dyslexia Project. I am keen to share with people what I have been through and to spread the message.

I had suffered so much growing up thinking that I was alone and my problems were unique. Now, wherever I go I'm stopped by people young and old, from all walks of life, who have gone through similar experiences. It's important for people to know they don't need to suffer alone. I hope that in publicising learning difficulties and the remarkable Dore Programme, the lives of others can be changed completely in the same way as my and my children's have.